Intermittent Fasting Success Manual

Eat, Fast, and Thrive: Your Guide to a Healthier You!

Donna Johnson

Copyright 2023-

Donna Johnson

ISBN

Printed in the United States of America

Disclaimer

This publication is designed to provide competent and reliable information regarding the subject covered However, the views expressed in this publication are those of the author alone and should not be taken as expert instruction or professional advice The reader is responsible for his or her actions The author hereby disclaims any responsibility or liability whatsoever that is incurred from the use or application of the contents of this publication by the purchaser of the reader. The purchaser or reader is hereby responsible for his or her actions.

All rights reserved. No part of this publication may be reproduced, distributed or transmitted in any form or by any means, including photocopying, recording or other electronic or mechanical methods without the prior written permission of the publisher except in the case of owner quotations embodied in critical reviews and certain other non-commercial uses permitted by copyright law For permission requests write to the publisher addressed at the address below

Table of Contents

INTRODUCTION

Thank you for visiting "Intermittent Fasting Success Manual." This book is your ticket to a life-changing journey to a healthier, slimmer, and more energetic you. If you've ever wanted to lose weight, improve your health, and enjoy delicious meals along the road, you've found your loyal partner.

In a world of fad diets and quick cures, intermittent fasting stands out as a refreshingly sensible and scientifically supported method to long-term weight reduction and general health improvement. It is not just about what you eat, but also about when you eat. Intermittent fasting takes use of the magic of time to enable your body to reset, regenerate, and enjoy extraordinary benefits.

This book is intended to serve as a complete guide, a coach, and a recipe book all in one. Whether you're new to intermittent fasting or want to fine-tune your approach, our goal is to offer you with the information, methods, and delectable recipes you need to make your fasting journey a delightful and victorious one.

What is the significance of "Leaner by the Hour"?

The idea behind "Leaner by the Hour" is simple yet effective. As you accept intermittent fasting, you're getting closer to becoming a slimmer, healthier version of yourself. This handbook isn't just about quick results; it's about long-term success. You'll discover how to take advantage of the 24-hour clock, reshaping your body and mind hour by hour, meal after meal.

CHAPTER ONE
BENEFITS BEYOND THE SCALE

Weight Loss

Weight Loss with Intermittent Fasting:

1. Caloric Restriction: Caloric restriction is one of the key processes behind weight reduction with intermittent fasting. You naturally minimize your total calorie consumption by restricting the time frame in which you eat calories. This calorie deficit is essential for weight reduction because it promotes the body to burn stored fat for energy, resulting in progressive and long-term weight loss.

2. Fat Burning: Insulin levels decrease while fasting, enabling your body to utilize stored fat for energy. This procedure, known as lipolysis, is highly successful in removing stubborn fat, particularly around the belly.

3. Metabolic Enhancement: Contrary to popular belief, intermittent fasting may actually enhance your metabolism. You increase insulin sensitivity and your body's capacity to manage blood sugar by cycling between fasting and feeding phases.

This metabolic flexibility may help with weight reduction and weight control in the long run.

4. Appetite Regulation: Fasting may aid in the regulation of appetite hormones like ghrelin and leptin. Many individuals discover that their cravings and general hunger diminish with time, making it simpler to regulate portion sizes and limit snacking, which contributes to weight reduction.

5. Lean Muscle Preservation: Intermittent fasting tends to retain lean muscle mass, owing to the fact that it prioritizes fat reserves for energy rather than breaking down muscle tissue. Maintaining a healthy body composition while decreasing weight is critical.

A Fountain of Health with Intermittent Fasting

1. Weight control: A key component of general wellness is weight control. Intermittent fasting aids in weight management by managing calorie intake, increasing fat loss, and maintaining lean muscle composition. Maintaining a healthy weight is critical for lowering the risk of a variety of health concerns, such as heart disease, diabetes, and joint difficulties.

2. Improved Insulin Sensitivity: Intermittent fasting improves insulin sensitivity, enabling cells to absorb and use glucose more effectively from the circulation. This impact is especially advantageous for those who have insulin resistance, prediabetes, or type 2 diabetes since it may help stabilize blood sugar levels and lessen the need for medication.

3. Heart Health: Intermittent fasting has been linked to better heart health. It can decrease blood pressure, lower "bad" LDL cholesterol and triglyceride levels, and raise "good" HDL cholesterol. These modifications lead to a lower risk of heart disease and its consequences.

4. Inflammation Reduction: Chronic inflammation is a role in a variety of health concerns, including autoimmune illnesses, cancer, and cardiovascular difficulties. Intermittent fasting has been demonstrated to lower inflammation indicators in the body, possibly lowering the risk of inflammatory illnesses.

5. Cellular Autophagy: Fasting activates an autophagy process in which cells remove damaged or malfunctioning components and recycle them. This cellular "clean-up" increases

cellular health and lifespan, which may lower the risk of age-related disorders.

6. Brain Health and Cognitive Function: Intermittent fasting may benefit brain health by increasing the synthesis of brain-derived neurotrophic factor (BDNF), a protein that promotes neuron development. This has the potential to improve cognitive performance, memory, and mood management.

7. Longevity: While further study is required, intermittent fasting seems to have the potential to increase lifetime. Fasting may help guard against the aging process and age-related disorders by increasing cellular repair and resilience.

8. Gut Health: Fasting intervals might give much-needed relaxation to the digestive system, possibly enhancing gut health. Some people report relief from digestive difficulties such as bloating, indigestion, and irritable bowel syndrome (IBS) symptoms.

9. Autonomic nerve System Balance: Intermittent fasting may aid in the balance of the autonomic nerve system, which regulates vital activities including heart rate, blood pressure, and

digestion. Obtaining this equilibrium may improve overall physiological resiliency.

10. Better Immune Function: Fasting may boost the immune system by increasing immune cell production and decreasing inflammation. This may boost the body's capacity to fight infections and diseases.

11. Emotional Well-Being: Some individuals experience enhanced emotional well-being when fasting, including less anxiety and greater stress resilience. Fasting as a regimen and discipline might have psychological benefits.

CHAPTER TWO

THE 16/8 METHOD

A Time-Restricted Feast

Intermittent fasting involves a variety of tactics, one of which is time-restricted food. This strategy is confining your daily food consumption to a set window of time, often 8-12 hours, while fasting for the other hours of the day or night. Here's a thorough description of the concept:

Fasting and Feasting Periods:

1. Fasting Window: You refrain from consuming calories during the fasting hours. Non-caloric drinks, such as water, tea, or black coffee, are OK. Depending on the procedure, this fasting phase might last anywhere from 12 to 16 hours or even more.

2. Feasting Window: The feasting window is the time period during which you eat all of your daily calories and meals. This window usually occurs within an 8-12 hour timeframe, enabling you to enjoy your meals while still meeting your nutritional demands.

Advantages of a Timed Feast:

1. Caloric Control: Restricting your meals to a certain time frame minimizes your calorie intake automatically. This calorie restriction is a critical component of weight control and fat reduction.

2. Increased Fat Burning: When you fast, your insulin levels decrease, encouraging your body to use stored fat for energy. This fat-burning mechanism, known as lipolysis, aids in weight reduction and body composition improvement.

3. Blood Sugar Regulation: Reducing the frequency of meals and snacks may help balance blood sugar levels. This is especially advantageous for those who have insulin resistance or are at risk of developing type 2 diabetes.

4. Metabolic Advantages: A time-limited feast may improve metabolic flexibility by increasing insulin sensitivity. This may result in improved blood sugar management and a lower risk of metabolic diseases.

5. Simplicity and Sustainability: When compared to more complicated fasting regimens, many people find time-restricted eating simpler to adopt into their everyday routines. This ease of use may encourage long-term adherence to the strategy.

6. Appetite Regulation: Some people notice increased appetite control and fewer cravings over time, making it simpler to stick to a balanced diet and portion sizes.

7. Digestive Rest: Fasting for an extended length of time gives the digestive system a rest, perhaps lowering digestive pain and increasing gut health.

Individualization and adaptability:

One of the benefits of time-restricted feasting is its flexibility to different tastes and lifestyles. You may choose the fasting and feasting times that are most convenient for your daily routine and personal preferences. People will find it simpler to implement intermittent fasting into their life as a result of this flexibility.

Potential Points to Consider:

1. Nutritional Quality: While time-restricted feasting does not mandate certain dietary choices, it is important to pay attention to the nutritional quality of your meals within the feasting window. Balanced, nutrient-dense meals are critical for good health.

2. Hydration: It is important to stay hydrated, particularly during fasting times. To avoid dehydration, drink lots of water or other non-caloric liquids.

Sample Meal Plans and Recipes

Meal Plan 1:

Fasting Hours (8:00 PM – 12:00 PM):

a. Drink plenty of water, herbal tea, or black coffee to stay hydrated.

Eating Hours (12:00 PM – 8:00 PM):

Lunch:

1. Grilled chicken breast on a bed of mixed greens with a vinaigrette dressing.

2. Quinoa salad with cucumbers, cherry tomatoes, and a lemon-tahini dressing.

Snack:

1. Greek yogurt with honey and fresh berries.

Dinner:

1. Baked salmon with garlic and roasted asparagus.
2. Brown rice or cauliflower rice, steamed.

Optional dessert: A tiny piece of dark chocolate (70% cocoa or higher).

Meal Plan 2:

Fasting Hours (7:00 p.m. to 11:00 a.m.):

a. Stay hydrated by drinking water, herbal tea, or black coffee.

Eating Hours (11:00 a.m. to 7:00 p.m.):

1. Scrambled eggs with spinach and feta cheese for brunch.
2. A piece of whole-grain toast or whole-grain bread.

Snack:

1. Cucumber and carrot sticks dipped in hummus.

Dinner:

1. Tofu or tempeh stir-fried with broccoli, bell peppers, and a ginger-soy sauce.
2. Quinoa or brown rice.

Optional snack: A small dish of mixed berries with whipped cream.

Meal Plan 3:

Fasting Hours (9:00 p.m. to 1:00 p.m.):

   a. Drink plenty of water, herbal tea, or black coffee to stay hydrated.

Eating Hours: 1:00 PM to 9:00 PM*

Lunch:

   1. Salad of chickpeas, cherry tomatoes, cucumber, red onion, and lemon-tahini dressing.
   2. Pita bread made from whole grains.

Snack: a handful of almonds or walnuts.

Dinner: Grilled shrimp with steamed broccoli and quinoa on the side.

Optional dessert: Greek yogurt parfait with layers of fruit and a sprinkle of honey.

Meal Plan 4:

Fasting Hours (8:00 PM – 12:00 PM):*

   a. Drink plenty of water, herbal tea, or black coffee to stay hydrated.

Eating Hours (12:00 PM – 8:00 PM):

Lunch: Lentil soup with mixed greens salad and balsamic vinaigrette.

Snack: Apple slices with almond butter.

Dinner: Roasted Brussels sprouts and sweet potatoes with baked chicken thighs.

Optional dessert: A bowl of frozen yogurt with fresh fruit.

CHAPTER THREE

THE EAT-STOP-EAT METHOD

24-Hour Fasting for Success

"24-Hour Fasting for Success" is a kind of intermittent fasting that entails avoiding calorie intake for a complete 24-hour period. In this detailed discussion, we'll look at the notion of 24-hour fasting, its possible advantages, how to perform it safely, and success recommendations.

1. Durability: During a 24-hour fast, you refrain from eating for the whole day, from one meal to the next. For example, if you complete supper at 7:00 p.m., you will not eat again until 7:00 p.m. the next day.

2. Water and Non-Caloric Drinks: It is critical to remain hydrated when fasting. During the fast, you may consume water, herbal tea, or black coffee with no additional sugar or cream. These drinks assist to satisfy hunger and keep you hydrated.

Benefits of 24-Hour Fasting:

1. Loss of Weight: A 24-hour fast results in a considerable calorie deficit, which may result in

long-term weight reduction. During the fast, the body depends mostly on stored fat for energy.

2. Metabolic Advantages: Intermittent fasting, especially 24-hour fasting, has been shown to increase insulin sensitivity and blood sugar levels, possibly lowering the risk of insulin resistance and type 2 diabetes.

3. Cellular Regeneration: Fasting over an extended length of time may activate autophagy, a process in which cells remove and recycle damaged components. This procedure aids in cellular repair and lifespan.

4. Simplicity: The 24-hour fasting method is very simple since it does not include extensive meal preparation or calorie tracking on non-fasting days.

5. Improved Appetite Control: Some people find that fasting for 24 hours on occasion helps them manage their appetite, eliminate cravings, and improve their portion control on non-fasting days.

Tips for Success with 24-Hour Fasting:

1. Plan your Fast: Select a day for your 24-hour fast that fits your schedule and lifestyle. Fasting on a

day when you have less social responsibilities and can concentrate on self-care may be simpler.

2. Stay Hydrated: Throughout the fasting phase, drink lots of water and non-caloric liquids to avoid dehydration and suppress hunger.

3. Get Busy: Do anything to get your mind off eating. Light exercise, reading, working, or engaging in hobbies may all help to keep hunger at bay.

4. Break your Fast Mindfully: To give lasting energy and minimize overeating, choose a balanced meal that contains protein, healthy fats, and fiber-rich carbs when it's time to break your fast.

5. Monitor Your Body: Keep track of how your body reacts to a 24-hour fast. If you suffer dizziness, weakness, or discomfort, it is critical that you listen to your body and, if necessary, break your fast.

6. Maintain Consistency: The key to obtaining the advantages of 24-hour fasting is consistency. To obtain and sustain the desired outcomes, repeat it on a regular basis, such as once or twice a week.

Warrior's Way to a Leaner You

In the context of intermittent fasting, the phrase "Warrior's Way to a Leaner You" refers to a particular fasting technique known as the Warrior Diet. This diet is distinguished by a longer fast followed by a shorter eating window.

Fasting Period (Undereating Period):

1. Extended Fasting Period: The Warrior Diet includes a lengthy fasting period of roughly 20 hours, known as the "undereating" phase. You eat few calories during this period, largely from non-caloric liquids such as water, herbal tea, or black coffee.

2. Catabolic Condition: This extended fasting period causes your body to enter a catabolic state, in which it largely uses stored fat for energy. This may help with weight loss and fat reduction.

3. Suppression of Appetite: Many people find that fasting for a considerable part of the day helps them regulate their hunger and lower their total calorie consumption.

Feasting Period (Overeating Period):

1. Limited Eating Period: The Warrior Diet has a brief eating window that lasts around 4 hours. This period is known as the "overeating" period.
2. Well-Rounded Meals: You eat your daily calorie intake in the form of balanced, nutrient-dense meals throughout the feasting window. Prioritizing entire foods, such as lean proteins, whole grains, fruits and vegetables, and healthy fats, is critical.
3. Satiety and Happiness: The focused eating window helps you to appreciate your meals, try new foods, and feel full on fewer, bigger meals.

Benefits of the Warrior Diet:

1. Weight Control: The fasting and feasting stages of the Warrior Diet produce a calorie deficit, which may contribute to weight loss and fat loss over time.
2. Improved Insulin Sensitivity: Intermittent fasting, such as the Warrior Diet, may improve insulin sensitivity, which may aid in blood sugar regulation and lower the development of insulin resistance.

3. Appetite Regulation: The fasting phase may improve better appetite control, lowering snacking frequency and calorie intake.

4. Fat Burning Acceleration: During the fasting period, the body depends on stored fat for energy, possibly speeding up fat burning.

5. Ease of Use: Because it incorporates fewer meals and snacks throughout the day, the structure of the Warrior Diet may make meal planning and calorie monitoring easier.

Tips for Success with the Warrior Diet:

1. Gradual Transition: If you're new to the Warrior Diet, try beginning with shorter fasting and feasting times and progressively increasing them.

2. Keep Hydrated: During the fasting phase, drink lots of water and non-caloric liquids to keep hydrated.

3. Balanced Meals: To satisfy your nutritional requirements, focus on balanced, nutrient-dense meals throughout the feasting window.

4. Mindful Eating: During the overeating period, practice mindful eating to relish your meals and avoid overindulgence.

Safety Considerations: The Warrior Diet may not be appropriate for everyone, particularly those with specific medical issues, pregnant or nursing women, or anyone with a history of eating disorders. When choosing fasting methods, always prioritize your health and well-being.

Warrior Approved Recipes

S/N	Warrior Approved Recipes	S/N	Warrior Approved Recipes
1	Grilled Chicken and Quinoa Bowl	2	Greek Yogurt Parfait
	- Grilled chicken breast seasoned with herbs and spices. Served with cooked quinoa. - Garnished with sautéed veggies (bell peppers, zucchini, and cherry tomatoes) and a sprinkle of olive oil.		- Greek yogurt layered with fresh berries (strawberries, blueberries, or raspberries). - For extra taste and texture, top with chopped nuts (almonds or walnuts) and a drizzle of honey.
3	Salmon and Asparagus Foil Packets	4	Quinoa and Chickpea Salad

	- Salmon fillets seasoned with lemon juice, garlic, and dill. - Served with fresh asparagus spears. - Wrapped in foil and cooked till tender.		- A substantial salad with cooked quinoa. - Tossed with chickpeas, sliced cucumber, cherry tomatoes, red onion, and fresh herbs. - Toss with a lemon-tahini dressing for a punch of flavor.
5	Stir-Fried Tofu and Broccoli	6	Mediterranean Hummus meal
	Cubes of tofu stir-fried with broccoli florets and a fragrant ginger-soy sauce, served over a bed of brown rice or cauliflower rice.		A Mediterranean-inspired meal with hummus, olives, cherry tomatoes, cucumber slices, and whole-grain pita bread. Ideal for creating and enjoying a variety of little snacks.
7	Protein-Packed Omelet	8	Tuna Salad Stuffed Avocado

	- A fluffy omelet stuffed with sautéed spinach, bell peppers, and chopped tomatoes. - To add flavor, top with feta cheese and fresh herbs.		- A creamy tuna salad prepared with canned tuna, Greek yogurt, celery, and seasonings. Served in half avocados for a healthful and full dinner.
9	Vegetable and Chickpea Curry		
	A tasty curry made with chickpeas, carrots, onions, and a combination of fragrant spices. Serve with brown rice or quinoa for a filling supper.		

CHAPTER FIVE

OMAD (ONE MEAL A DAY)

The Ultimate Fast

"The Ultimate Fast" usually refers to a long fast, frequently lasting 36 hours or more. This fasting strategy goes beyond typical intermittent fasting approaches such as the 16/8 or Warrior Diet, which have shorter fasting times.

1. Extended Fasting time: Compared to other intermittent fasting regimens, "The Ultimate Fast" requires a much longer fasting time. This fasting phase often lasts 36 hours or longer, implying that you refrain from calorie ingestion for a lengthy period of time.

2. Flexible Structure: While "The Ultimate Fast" normally entails a time of continuous fasting, there is some leeway in how it is carried out. Some varieties allow for a certain amount of calorie intake throughout the fasting period, generally in the form of non-caloric liquids, but others encourage full calorie abstinence.

Potential Benefits of "The Ultimate Fast:

1. Increased Fat Burning: With a longer fast, the body has more time to deplete glycogen reserves and enter ketosis, when it predominantly depends on stored fat for energy. This may hasten fat loss.
2. Autophagy in Cells: Prolonged fasting may activate autophagy, a cellular mechanism in which the body eliminates and recycles damaged components, increasing cellular repair and lifespan.
3. Sensitivity to Insulin: Fasting over an extended period of time may enhance insulin sensitivity and help manage blood sugar levels, both of which are helpful to overall metabolic health.
4. Appetite Regulation: Some people find that fasting for prolonged periods of time helps to manage their appetite and lessen cravings, perhaps leading to improved calorie control.
5. Simplicity: "The Ultimate Fast" may reduce meal preparation time and remove the need for several meals and snacks throughout the day.

Considerations for "The Ultimate Fast:

1. Hydration: It is critical to stay hydrated when fasting for a lengthy period of time. To avoid dehydration, drink lots of water and non-caloric liquids.

2. Electrolytes: If your fasting period exceeds 36 hours, consider supplementing with electrolytes such as salt, potassium, and magnesium. This may aid with electrolyte balance.

3. Personal Tolerance: Fasting over a lengthy period of time is not for everyone. Some people may feel pain, weariness, dizziness, or other negative symptoms. Always pay attention to your body and make necessary adjustments.

4. Refeeding: When breaking a lengthy fast, reintroduce modest, readily digested meals. Avoid overindulging since your stomach may have shrunk during the fast.

Safety Precautions:

1. Prioritize safety and watch your body's reaction throughout "The Ultimate Fast." Break the fast and seek medical treatment if you feel extreme pain or unpleasant consequences.

2. "The Ultimate Fast" should not be done on a regular basis. It's usually done on a regular basis,

such as once a month or on occasion, to minimize the possible harmful health implications of extended fasting.

Tantalizing OMAD Recipes

S/N	Tantalizing OMAD Recipes	S/N	Tantalizing OMAD Recipes
10	Skewers of grilled steak and vegetables	11	Mediterranean Chickpea Salad
	Served with quinoa or baked sweet potato and skewers of marinated beef cubes with colorful bell peppers, onions, and zucchini.		A filling salad of chickpeas, cucumbers, cherry tomatoes, red onions, and Kalamata olives. Tossed with a lemon-tahini vinaigrette, with crumbled feta cheese and fresh parsley on top.
12	Lemon-Dill Baked Salmon	13	Thai Chicken and Vegetable Stir-Fry

	Baked salmon fillet seasoned with dill, lemon zest, and garlic. - Drizzled with a creamy Greek yogurt and lemon sauce. With steamed broccoli or asparagus on the side.		Chicken breast slices stir-fried with colorful bell peppers, snap peas, and carrots in a handmade Thai-inspired sauce prepared with coconut milk, ginger, and chili paste. Served with cauliflower or brown rice.
14	Portobello Mushrooms Stuffed with Caprese	15	Stuffed Spinach and Feta Chicken Breast
	Stuffed Portobello mushrooms with chopped tomatoes, fresh mozzarella cheese, and basil leaves. Baked until the cheese is melty and golden, then drizzled with balsamic glaze.		Stuffed chicken breasts with sautéed spinach, crumbled feta cheese, and garlic; baked to perfection and served with roasted asparagus or a mixed green salad.
16	Quinoa and Black Bean Bowl	17	Moroccan-Spiced Lamb Tagine

	- Made with cooked quinoa and topped with black beans, corn, diced avocado, and diced tomatoes. - Fresh cilantro and a sprinkle of lime-tahini dressing finish the dish.		Slow-cooked lamb tagine with Moroccan spices, dried fruits, and vegetables; served with couscous or cauliflower couscous as a side.
18	Thai Green Curry with Tofu and Vegetables	19	Salad with Shrimp and Avocado
	- Tofu cubes with assorted veggies (e.g., bell peppers, eggplant, and snow peas) cooked in a fragrant Thai green curry sauce. - Served with rice noodles or jasmine rice.		- A light salad made with cooked shrimp, avocado slices, cherry tomatoes, and cucumber. - Dressed with a tangy lime-cilantro vinaigrette.
20	Stuffed Bell Peppers with Roasted Vegetables and Quinoa		
	Stuffed bell peppers with roasted veggies,		

| cooked quinoa, and feta cheese. Bake until the peppers are soft and the filling is well cooked. | | |

CHAPTER SIX

TASTY RECIPES FOR SUCCESS

Breakfast Bites

S/N	Breakfast Bites	S/N	Breakfast Bites
21	Peanut Butter Banana Oatmeal	22	Almond Date Energy
	- A mixture of rolled oats, mashed bananas, natural peanut butter, and honey. - Form into bite-sized balls and place in the refrigerator until solid.		- In a food processor, combine almonds, pitted dates, cinnamon, and vanilla essence until a sticky dough forms. - Refrigerate tiny balls of dough.
23	Mini Vegetable Frittatas	24	Chia Pudding
	- In a mixing bowl, combine eggs and your choice of chopped veggies (e.g., bell peppers, spinach, onions). - Fill tiny muffin cups halfway with batter and bake until set.		Combine chia seeds, almond milk, maple syrup, and vanilla essence. Fill little silicone molds halfway with the mixture and freeze until hard.

25	Mini Spinach and Feta Quiches	26	Blueberry Protein
	Whisk together the eggs, chopped spinach, crumbled feta cheese, and nutmeg. Fill tiny muffin cups halfway with batter and bake until golden.		Combine rolled oats, protein powder, almond butter, and dried blueberries in a mixing bowl. - Roll into tiny bits and chill.
27	Sweet Potato Breakfast	28	Chocolate Avocado Truffles
	Mash cooked sweet potatoes with eggs, cinnamon, and honey to taste. Spoon into tiny muffin pans and bake until done.		Combine ripe avocado, chocolate powder, honey, and vanilla essence; shape into little truffles and refrigerate.
29	Breakfast Muffins with Ham and Cheese	30	Raspberry Almond Breakfast
	- Line muffin cups with slices of lean ham to form a "crust." - Layer scrambled eggs, chopped bell		- Mix together almond flour, frozen raspberries, and honey.

peppers, and shredded cheese on top. Bake until the cheese is melted.		- Shape into bite-sized balls and chill.	

Lunchtime Delights

S/N	Lunchtime Delights	S/N	Lunchtime Delights
31	Salad with grilled chicken and balsamic vinaigrette	32	Mediterranean Hummus Wrap
	Grilled chicken breast slices over a bed of mixed greens, cherry tomatoes, cucumber, and red onion with a homemade balsamic vinaigrette dressing.		A whole-grain tortilla stuffed with hummus, cucumber slices, cherry tomatoes, Kalamata olives, and feta cheese. Roll it up and eat it.
33	Thai Tofu and Vegetable Stir-Fry	34	Caprese Quinoa Salad
	Stir-fried tofu slices with colorful bell peppers, snap peas, and carrots in a handmade Thai-inspired sauce prepared with coconut milk, ginger, and chili paste.		Quinoa cooked with cherry tomatoes, fresh mozzarella cheese, basil leaves, and drizzled with balsamic sauce.

	- Served with cauliflower or brown rice.		
35	Salad with Chickpeas and Avocado	36	Soup with lentils and vegetables
	A light salad tossed in a lime-tahini dressing with chickpeas, sliced avocado, red onion, and cilantro.		A substantial soup seasoned with herbs and spices and cooked with lentils, sliced carrots, celery, and spinach.
37	Stuffed Portobello Mushrooms with Spinach and Feta	38	Thai Coconut Curry Noodle Bowl
	Stuffed Portobello mushrooms with sautéed spinach, crumbled feta cheese, and garlic; baked until soft.		Rice noodles with tofu or shrimp in a creamy coconut curry sauce. - Garnish with fresh cilantro and lime wedges.
39	Greek Chicken Pita Pocket	40	Stuffed Bell Peppers with Salmon and Quinoa
	Grilled chicken strips in a whole-wheat pita pocket. Add chopped cucumbers,		Baked until peppers are soft, then packed with cooked quinoa, flaked salmon,

S/N		S/N	
	tomatoes, red onions, and tzatziki sauce to taste.		chopped tomatoes, and dill.
41	Stuffed Spinach and Artichoke Chicken Breast	42	Lettuce Wraps with Avocado and Turkey
	Baked chicken breasts with sautéed spinach, artichoke hearts, and cream cheese until chicken is cooked through.		Large lettuce leaves stuffed with sliced turkey, mashed avocado, chopped tomatoes, and a balsamic glaze drizzle.
43	Tagine de Chickpeas et Vegetables Marocaine		
	A delicious tagine made with chickpeas, veggies, and Moroccan spices. Served with couscous or cauliflower couscous as a side dish.		

Dinner Delicacies

S/N	Dinner Delicacies	S/N	Dinner Delicacies

44	Grilled Salmon with Lemon-Dill Sauce	45	Spaghetti Squash with Pesto and Cherry Tomatoes
	Sprinkle dill, lemon zest, and garlic over salmon fillets. Grill until done, then top with a creamy Greek yogurt and lemon sauce.		- Roast the spaghetti squash until cooked, then scrape the threads out. - Toss with halved cherry tomatoes and homemade basil pesto.
46	Salad with grilled vegetables and quinoa	47	Stir-Fry with Chicken and Vegetables
	- Grill a variety of veggies (eggplant, bell peppers, zucchini) and combine with cooked quinoa. - Garnish with fresh herbs and drizzle with balsamic vinaigrette.		- Cook chicken strips with colorful bell peppers, broccoli florets, and snap peas in a skillet. - Serve with brown rice or cauliflower rice and a homemade stir-fry sauce.
48	Parmesan Eggplant	49	Cauliflower and Chickpea Curry
	- Baked eggplant slices covered with		Aromatic curry with cauliflower florets,

	breadcrumbs and Parmesan cheese till golden. - Bake until bubbling, then layer with marinara sauce and mozzarella cheese.		chickpeas, and a spice combination. With basmati rice or whole-grain naan bread, serve.
50	Stuffed Bell Peppers with Turkey and Quinoa	51	Stir-Fry of Beef and Broccoli
	Baked until peppers are soft with a combination of ground turkey, cooked quinoa, diced tomatoes, and spices.		Stir-fried sliced beef with broccoli florets in a delicious garlic ginger sauce. Over brown rice or cauliflower rice, serve.
52	Mediterranean Shrimp with Quinoa	53	Sweet Potato and Black Bean Chili
	Cook shrimp with garlic, cherry tomatoes, Kalamata olives, and feta cheese in a skillet. Drizzle with olive oil and serve over cooked quinoa.		Sweet potatoes, black beans, chopped tomatoes, and chili spices combine to make a hearty chili. Simmer until the flavors combine.

54	Spinach and Feta Stuffed Chicken Breast	55	Vegan Lentil and Vegetable Curry
	Sautéed spinach, crumbled feta cheese, and garlic fill chicken breasts; bake until chicken is cooked through.		A vegan curry made with red lentils, a variety of veggies, and coconut milk. Serve with naan bread or jasmine rice.
56	Teriyaki Tofu and Vegetable Stir-Fry	57	Lemon Herb Grilled Chicken
	Stir-fried tofu cubes with colorful bell peppers, snap peas, and carrots. Serve with brown rice or cauliflower rice with a homemade teriyaki sauce.		Marinate chicken breasts in a lemon juice, herb, and olive oil combination. Grill until done and serve with roasted veggies on the side.

Snacks and Treats

S/N	Snacks & Treats	S/N	Snacks & Treats
58	Hummus and vegetable sticks	59	Almond Butter with Banana Slices
	Serve with carrot sticks, cucumber slices, and bell		For a filling and naturally sweet snack, spread almond butter over banana slices.

	pepper strips for dipping.		
60	Trail Mix	61	Pineapple Cottage Cheese
	For a balanced snack, combine unsalted nuts, dried fruits (e.g., raisins, apricots), and dark chocolate chips.		For a protein-rich and refreshing treat, top a dish of cottage cheese with chopped pineapple.
62	Avocado and Tomato Rice Cakes	63	Chocolate Protein Balls
	Spread mashed avocado over rice cakes, then top with sliced tomatoes, salt & pepper, and balsamic glaze.		Combine protein powder, almond butter, honey, and cocoa powder in a mixing bowl. Refrigerate tiny balls of dough.
64	Frozen Grapes	65	Sea Salt Edamame
	Freeze grapes for a delicious, refreshing snack with a satisfying crunch.		For a high-protein, fiber-rich snack, steam edamame and season with sea salt.
66	Pineapple with Cottage Cheese	67	Almond Butter Apple Slices

	For a sweet and salty combo, combine cottage cheese with chopped pineapple.		For a pleasant and crispy snack, slice apples and dip them in almond butter.
68	Guacamole and vegetable dippers	69	Smoothie with Berries and Spinach
	Serve with sliced bell peppers, cherry tomatoes, and jicama sticks for dipping.		For a refreshing smoothie, combine berries (strawberries, blueberries), spinach, Greek yogurt, and a pinch of honey.
70	Roll-ups with cucumber and cream cheese	71	Almonds with Dark Chocolate Coating
	To make a crispy and creamy snack, spread cream cheese over cucumber slices and wrap them up.		Melt dark chocolate and coat almonds with it. Allow them to cool and solidify before serving.
72	Kale Chips		
	- Toss kale leaves with olive oil and spices of your choosing (e.g., salt, nutritional yeast).		

S/N			
	- Bake till golden brown.		

Satisfying Sweets

S/N	Satisfying Sweets	S/N	Satisfying Sweets
73	Greek Yogurt with Berries and Honey	74	Chocolate Avocado Mousse
	Drizzle honey over a bowl of Greek yogurt and top with fresh berries (e.g., blueberries, strawberries, raspberries).		For a velvety and healthful chocolate mousse, combine ripe avocado, cocoa powder, honey, and vanilla essence.
75	Frozen Banana Bites	76	Chia Seed Pudding
	Cut bananas into bite-sized rounds, then dip them in melted dark chocolate and place in the freezer until hardened.		Combine chia seeds, almond milk, maple syrup, and vanilla essence in a mixing bowl. - Refrigerate until the liquid thickens, then top with fresh fruit.
77	Mixed Berry Sorbet:	78	Baked Apple Cinnamon Oatmeal Cups
	- Blend together frozen berries and		Combine rolled oats, chopped apples,

	honey or agave syrup until smooth. - Serve immediately for a cool sorbet.		cinnamon, and honey to taste. Bake in muffin cups until golden brown.
79	Dark Chocolate-Dipped Strawberries	80	Cinnamon-Baked Apples
	- Melt dark chocolate and dip in fresh strawberries. - Allow to cool and solidify before serving.		- Core the apples and sprinkle with cinnamon and brown sugar. - Serve with a dollop of Greek yogurt after baking until soft.
81	Berry-Yogurt Parfait	82	Mini Banana Nut Muffins
	For a pleasant and sweet treat, layer vanilla yogurt with mixed berries and granola.		Use ripe bananas, chopped almonds, and whole wheat flour to make tiny muffins that may be sweetened with honey or maple syrup.
83	Protein Balls with Peanut Butter and Chocolate	84	Oatmeal Raisin Cookies
	Combine protein powder, peanut		To add sweetness, bake oatmeal cookies

	butter, chocolate powder, and honey to taste. Refrigerate tiny balls of dough.		with raisins, cinnamon, and a drizzle of honey.
85	Fruit Salad with Mint-Lime Dressing	86	Chocolate Almond Butter Cups
	Toss fresh fruits (such as melon, berries, and citrus) with a dressing consisting of fresh lime juice and chopped mint leaves.		- Melt dark chocolate and spoon some into tiny muffin liners. - Top with a dollop of almond butter and extra melted chocolate. - Refrigerate until firm.
87	Pumpkin Pie Energy Bites	88	Mango Coconut Sorbet
	Combine pumpkin puree, oats, pumpkin spice, and honey. Refrigerate after rolling into little bits.		- Combine mango chunks, coconut milk, and honey in a blender. - For a tropical sorbet, freeze until firm.

CHAPTER SEVEN
COMBINING INTERMITTENT FASTING WITH EXERCISE

Fitness for Fasters

"Fitness for Fasters" refers to exercise and physical activity techniques that persons who practice intermittent fasting may use to improve their general health, fitness levels, and accomplish their health objectives more efficiently. Intermittent fasting may be paired with a variety of workout regimens to get the best outcomes. Here is a full discussion of fitness issues for persons who practice intermittent fasting:

Exercise Timing:

1. Quick Workouts: Some people prefer to exercise during their fasting window, which is usually in the morning. Because glycogen levels are depleted following an overnight fast, this strategy may boost fat burning. It is, however, critical to ensure that you have adequate energy and fluids during the activity.

2. Fed Exercises: Others would rather exercise within their meal window in order to get more nutrition and energy. This method may be useful

for high-intensity exercises that need more energy.

Exercise Types:

1. Aerobic (Cardiovascular) Exercise: Jogging, cycling, swimming, and brisk walking may all help you lose weight and improve your cardiovascular health. Depending on personal taste, either fasted or fed cardio may be successful.

2. Strength Training (Resistance Exercise): Resistance training, which includes weightlifting and bodyweight exercises, aids in the development of muscle mass and the stimulation of metabolism. It is possible to do it during fasting or eating windows.

3. HIIT (High-Intensity Interval Training): Short bursts of intensive activity are followed by brief rest intervals in HIIT exercises. These are fat-burning exercises that may be done throughout fasting or eating periods.

4. Training for Flexibility and Mobility: Stretching and yoga activities may increase flexibility and lower the chance of injury. These workouts may be done whenever you choose.

Hydration: It is critical to stay hydrated, particularly while exercising during fasting times. To avoid dehydration, drink water or non-caloric drinks.

Nutrition Prior to Exercise: If you prefer to exercise during your fasting period, consume a modest, balanced meal or snack before your activity to ensure you have enough energy and nutrition. This might include glucose and protein sources.

Nutrition Post-Workout: Following your exercise, concentrate on replenishing nutrients and boosting healing. A well-balanced breakfast or snack including protein, carbs, and healthy fats may help with muscle regeneration and glycogen replenishment.

Pay Attention to Your Body: Pay attention to your body's signals and make any adjustments to your workout plan. If fasting exercises make you feel tired or disoriented, it may be advisable to exercise within your eating window.

Consistency is Essential: Maintaining consistency in your workout program is essential for long-term success. Find an exercise routine and a fasting plan that work for your lifestyle and interests.

Recuperation and Rest: Get enough rest and prioritize your recuperation. This involves getting adequate sleep and giving your body enough time to recuperate between strenuous activities.

Changes over Time: As your body adjusts to intermittent fasting and exercise, you may need to change your regimen to experience continued success. Modifying the time and intensity of exercises is one example.

Benefits of Fasting-Friendly Exercise:
1. Increased Fat Burning: Exercising during fasting times may increase fat burning by using energy from stored fat.
2. Improved Insulin Sensitivity: Exercise, particularly cardiovascular and resistance training, may improve insulin sensitivity, which can supplement fasting's metabolic effects.
3. Hunger manage: Some people find that fasting-friendly activity helps them manage their hunger and cravings, making it simpler to stick to fasting regimens.
4. Stress Reduction: Activities such as yoga and Pilates encourage relaxation and stress reduction, which may be especially beneficial while fasting.

Tips for Fasting-Friendly Exercise:

1. Stay Hydrated: To avoid dehydration, drink water or non-caloric drinks before and throughout your exercise. Hydration is critical during fasting times.

2. Timing Is Everything: The best time to exercise while fasting differs from person to person. Some individuals like to exercise in the morning before breaking their fast, while others prefer to exercise later in the day.

3. Pay Attention to Your Body: Pay attention to how your body reacts to exercise while fasting. If you feel dizzy, weak, or uncomfortable, you should stop or adjust your exercise.

4. Modify Intensity: Lower-intensity exercises are often tolerated better during fasting times. Save your high-intensity exercises for when you have more energy and nutrients available for recuperation.

5. Post-Workout Nutrition: Prioritize a balanced meal with protein, carbs, and healthy fats after exercising while fasting to help muscle healing and energy replenishment.

Safety Considerations: If you are new to fasting or exercising while fasting, begin with shorter periods and gradually increase as your body adjusts.

Be alert of overexertion and dehydration symptoms, and always prioritize your safety and well-being.

CHAPTER EIGHT
OVERCOMING HURDLES

Managing Hunger and Cravings

1. Recognize the Hunger-Satiety Cycle: Hunger is a normal and recurring experience. It comes and goes in ebbs and flows. Recognize that if you give it some time, the first sense of hunger will usually go away.

2. Select the Appropriate Fasting Period: Choose an intermittent fasting technique that fits your lifestyle and natural hunger patterns. Some individuals like to fast at certain times of the day, while others prefer overnight fasting.

3. Maintain Hydration: Dehydration is frequently confused with appetite. During fasting hours, drink lots of water, herbal tea, or black coffee to keep hydrated and avoid false hunger signals.

4. Select Non-Caloric Beverages: During fasting, coffee and tea (without added sugar or cream) might help decrease hunger and offer a sensation of fullness.

5. Extend Your Fasting Period Gradually: If you're new to intermittent fasting, start with shorter

fasting windows and gradually increase them as your body adjusts.

6. Eat Fiber-Rich Foods: Fiber promotes satiety and may be ingested throughout mealtimes. Include veggies, fruits, healthy grains, and legumes in your meals to feel fuller for longer.

7. Put protein and healthy fats first: Protein and healthy fats satisfy more than carbs. Include lean protein sources like chicken, fish, tofu, and lentils in your meals, as well as healthy fats like avocados, almonds, and olive oil.

8. Prepare Balanced Meals: Make sure your meals are well-balanced and include a variety of macronutrients (protein, carbs, and fats) to give sustained energy and lower the chance of post-meal cravings.

9. Stress Management: Emotional eating and cravings may be triggered by stress. Incorporate stress-reduction practices into your regular routine, such as meditation, yoga, or deep breathing exercises.

10. Ways to Distract Yourself: When cravings occur, do something that gets your mind off eating. This might be taking a stroll, reading, or pursuing a hobby.

11. Make Use of Condiments and Spices: Flavorful condiments and spices may enhance the enjoyment and satisfaction of your meals. To add flavor without adding calories, experiment with herbs, spices, spicy sauce, or vinegar.

12. Engage in Mindful Eating: Focus on the sensory sensation of eating. Chew carefully, taste each mouthful, and pay attention throughout meals. This may assist you in identifying actual hunger and fullness signals.

13. Allow for Occasional Treats: It is OK to indulge in occasional indulgences or favorite meals within your eating window. Excessive self-restraint might lead to increased desires and overeating.

14. Get Enough Sleep: Sleep deprivation may interfere with hunger-regulating hormones and increase cravings. Each night, aim for 7-9 hours of decent sleep.

15. Be Consistent and Patient: Your body may need time to acclimate to intermittent fasting. Be gentle with yourself while adhering to your fasting routine.

Handling Social Situations

1. Share Your Fasting Schedule: Inform close friends and family about your intermittent fasting strategy. Explain your fasting schedule and why you picked this method. This might assist to minimize misconceptions and eating pressure during fasting times.

2. Selecting Social Events Wisely: Choose your social engagements carefully, particularly if they entail excessive or unhealthy food intake. Prioritize occasions that coincide with your fasting window or where you can eat healthily.

3. Make an offer to bring a dish: If you're going to a potluck or party, volunteer to bring a dish that corresponds to your nutritional choices and fasting schedule. This manner, you'll have a meal selection that you're comfortable eating.

4. Concentrate on Non-Food Activities: Suggest non-food-related social activities, such as going for a stroll, playing games, or sharing a hobby. This may assist to divert attention away from eating.

5. Watch Your Alcohol Consumption: If you choose to drink alcohol during your meal window, do so

sparingly. Alcohol may weaken inhibitions, causing overeating or bad dietary choices.

6. Make a Fasting Day Schedule: When fasting, organize your answers to food offers ahead of time. Explain that you are presently fasting and politely reject. Offer to help with non-food components of the social gathering.

7. Maintain Hydration: Keep a non-caloric beverage on hand for social engagements, such as water or herbal tea, to keep hydrated and to reduce hunger.

8. Refrain from Peer Pressure: Be prepared to be encouraged to break your fast by well-meaning friends or family members. Refuse politely and remind them of your commitment.

9. Get Ready for Food Temptations: If you anticipate temptations during social occasions, remind yourself of your intermittent fasting objectives and motives. Visualize the wonderful results you want.

10. Practice Adaptability: You may need to change your fasting schedule from time to time to satisfy social engagements. Remember that flexibility is key, and skipping a fasting day every now and then is not considered a failure.

11. Don't Be Hard on Yourself: If you depart from your fasting plan at a social function, don't beat yourself up over it. Recognize the lapse, learn from it, and resume your fasting regimen the following day.

Dealing with Side Effects

Intermittent fasting, like any dietary or lifestyle modification, may have unintended consequences. While many people benefit from intermittent fasting, certain individuals may have temporary difficulties. Here's a detailed description of how to cope with adverse effects while fasting intermittently:

1. Recognize Common Adverse Reactions: Recognize that adverse effects are frequent throughout the intermittent fasting adjustment period. Hunger, irritability, weariness, and cravings are common adverse effects.

2. Gradual Modification: Begin by introducing intermittent fasting gradually. Allow your body to adjust more smoothly to longer fasting windows or longer durations of fasting.

3. Maintain Hydration: Dehydration might worsen negative effects. Drink plenty of water, herbal tea,

or black coffee (no added sugar or cream) to keep hydrated during fasting hours.

4. Select Nutrient-Rich Foods: During your eating windows, choose nutrient-dense meals. Whole meals rich in vitamins, minerals, and fiber may help reduce adverse effects and promote general health.

5. Macronutrient Balance: Incorporate a variety of macronutrients (protein, carbs, and fats) into your meals to assist control energy levels and avoid severe hunger or cravings.

6. Stress Management: Stress might exacerbate negative effects. To alleviate stress, try stress-reduction strategies like meditation, yoga, or deep breathing exercises.

7. Pay Attention to Your Body: Be aware of hunger signals and how your body reacts to fasting. It's OK to change your fasting schedule or break your fast early if you're feeling very hungry or ill.

8. Make Use of Fasting Variations: Experiment with various intermittent fasting techniques. Certain versions, such as the 16/8 approach or the 5:2 diet, may be more suited to a person's tolerance to adverse effects.

9. Deal with Low Blood Sugar: If you have low blood sugar symptoms (hypoglycemia), such as dizziness or shakiness, break your fast with a modest, balanced snack including protein and carbs.

10. Electrolytes should be included: Include electrolyte-rich foods and drinks, such as salt, potassium, and magnesium, in your meals to assist maintain electrolyte balance.

11. Get Enough Sleep: Get enough sleep, since exhaustion and mood swings may be compounded by a lack of sleep. Each night, aim for 7-9 hours of decent sleep.

12. Gradually Introduce Exercise: If you're new to exercising, start slowly during your eating windows. Excessive effort might exacerbate adverse effects.

13. Be Patient: Recognize that side effects are often transient and may improve as your body adjusts to intermittent fasting. Allow yourself time to adapt and be patient.

14. Alter Your Approach: If you routinely experience unpleasant side effects from intermittent fasting, it may not be the best option for you. Prioritizing your entire health and well-being is critical.

15. Maintain a Journal: Keep a diary to document your side effects, meals, and fasting progress. This might assist you in identifying trends and making required changes.

CHAPTER NINE
LONG-TERM HEALTH AND WELLNESS

Preventing Weight Rebound

Preventing weight gain after reaching your goal weight using intermittent fasting is critical to long-term success. Weight rebound, often known as yo-yo dieting, happens when people recover weight after stopping a diet or fasting practice. Follow these thorough tactics to minimize weight regain when practicing intermittent fasting:

1. Transition from Fasting to Maintenance: Don't quit fasting suddenly after you've accomplished your desired weight or health objectives via intermittent fasting. Gradually transition from your fasting habit to a maintenance diet that includes frequent, balanced meals.

2. Establish Realistic Maintenance Objectives: Set reasonable weight maintenance goals that allow for minor variations. Rather of striving to remain at a certain weight, aim to stay within a fair range.

3. Determine Your Maintenance Calories: Calculate your maintenance calorie consumption

depending on your age, amount of exercise, and metabolism. This will give you an idea of how many calories you should take in order to maintain your present weight.

4. Keep Track of Your Caloric Intake: Monitor your calorie intake even when on maintenance. Continue to monitor your meals to ensure that you are not overdoing or underestimating your calorie intake.

5. Highlight Nutrient-Dense Foods: Eat nutrient-dense foods such as fruits, vegetables, lean meats, whole grains, and healthy fats. These meals give necessary nutrients and aid with hunger management.

6. Avoid Excessive Caloric Restriction: Avoid dramatically cutting your calorie intake once you've finished fasting. Extremely low-calorie diets may cause metabolic slowing and weight gain.

7. Maintain Physical Activity: Maintain a regular level of physical exercise. Exercise helps you burn calories, develop muscle, and maintain a healthy metabolism, which are all important for weight management.

8. Strength Training: Include strength training in your fitness regimen. Lean muscle mass may aid increase metabolism and enhance body composition.

9. Regularly monitor your weight: Track your weight on a regular basis to notice any big swings early on. This gives you the ability to take remedial action if necessary.

10. Refrain from Emotional Eating: Be aware of emotional eating. If you find yourself resorting to food for comfort, stress relief, or boredom, look for healthy coping techniques such as meditation, hobbies, or consulting with a therapist.

11. Stress Management: Excessive stress might cause weight gain. To keep stress at bay, use stress-reduction strategies such as meditation, yoga, or deep breathing exercises.

12. Get Enough Sleep: Make sleep a priority since it is important for weight management. To maintain general health, aim for 7-9 hours of quality sleep every night.

13. Maintain Hydration: Stay hydrated throughout the day. Thirst is often mistaken for hunger, resulting in needless calorie intake.

14. Meal Preparation and Planning: Plan and prepare your meals ahead of time. The availability of healthy, balanced meals lessens the temptation to make bad eating choices.

15. Be Patient and Realistic: Recognize that slight weight changes are natural. Prioritize long-term health and well-being above short-term metrics.

16. Maintain Your Commitment to Healthy Habits: Maintain the good behaviors you established throughout your fasting adventure. The key to avoiding weight rebound is consistency.

Anti-Aging Benefits Unveiled

In recent years, intermittent fasting has received attention for its possible anti-aging advantages, which include delaying the aging process and improving lifespan. While research is still underway, multiple pathways imply that intermittent fasting may have anti-aging benefits. Here's a detailed description of intermittent fasting's anti-aging benefits:

1. Autophagy and Cellular Repair: Autophagy, a cellular process that includes the elimination of damaged or defective cellular components, is one of the major processes behind intermittent fasting's anti-aging advantages. Fasting activates

autophagy, which allows cells to cleanse and repair themselves more efficiently. This mechanism may aid in the maintenance of cellular health and the reduction of the buildup of damaged components over time.

2. Oxidative Stress Reduction: Oxidative stress, induced by the buildup of damaging free radicals, is a major contributor to aging and age-related disorders. Intermittent fasting may lower oxidative stress by strengthening the body's antioxidant defenses and increasing the efficiency of mitochondria, the energy-producing components of the cell. Reduced oxidative stress may help protect cells and reduce the aging process.

3. Increased Insulin Sensitivity: Intermittent fasting may improve insulin sensitivity, which is important for blood sugar regulation. Improved insulin sensitivity lowers the risk of type 2 diabetes and metabolic syndrome, both of which are often linked to hastened aging.

4. Hormone Control: Fasting may affect hormone synthesis, particularly growth hormone and insulin-like growth factor 1 (IGF-1). These hormones are critical for development and aging.

Intermittent fasting may assist in optimizing their levels to promote healthy aging.

5. Activation of Longevity Genes: Intermittent fasting has been shown to activate certain genes linked to lifespan and cellular defense. SIRT1 and FOXO, for example, are involved in repairing DNA damage, enhancing stress tolerance, and prolonging lifespan.

6. Weight Control: A healthy weight is essential for anti-aging. Intermittent fasting may help with weight loss by encouraging calorie control and lowering the risk of obesity, which has been linked to accelerate aging and age-related disorders.

7. Brain Function: Fasting may benefit brain health by increasing the synthesis of brain-derived neurotrophic factor (BDNF), a protein that supports neuron development and maintenance. Improved brain function may contribute to cognitive vigor as people age.

8. Inflammation Reduction: Chronic inflammation is a defining feature of aging and age-related illnesses. Intermittent fasting has been found to lower inflammatory indicators, possibly decreasing the aging process and lowering the risk of chronic illnesses.

9. Disease Control: Intermittent fasting may lower the risk of age-related disorders such as heart disease, cancer, and neurological problems by increasing metabolic health, insulin sensitivity, and other variables.

10. Increased Cellular Resilience: By exposing cells to modest stress during fasting periods, intermittent fasting may improve cellular resilience. This stress causes cells to adapt and grow more resilient, which may have anti-aging benefits in the long run.

11. Better Immune Function: According to some research, intermittent fasting may improve the immune system's capacity to fight infections and disorders, hence improving general health and lifespan.

12. Adaptability in Lifestyle: Intermittent fasting is adaptable to different periods of life and circumstances, making it a potentially lifelong anti-aging strategy. It is adaptable to changing demands and tastes as people age.

CONCLUSION

FREQUENTLY ASKED QUESTIONS

Busting Fasting Myths

Intermittent fasting is becoming more popular as a dietary and lifestyle strategy for a variety of health advantages. However, as its popularity has grown, various myths and misunderstandings have evolved. To give accurate information regarding intermittent fasting, it is critical to address and refute these fallacies. Here's a detailed breakdown of some typical fasting myths:

1. Fasting Equals Starvation: Fasting is a purposeful and regulated practice of refraining from eating for a certain amount of time. It is not the same as starvation, which happens when the body is deprived of critical nutrients for a lengthy period of time. Intermittent fasting consists of planned fasting intervals followed by eating windows to ensure adequate nutrition intake during feeding hours.

2. Fasting Reduces Metabolism: Intermittent fasting may increase metabolism by improving insulin sensitivity and encouraging the body to utilize stored fat for energy. When done appropriately,

short-term fasting does not result in a substantial drop in metabolic rate.

3. Fasting causes muscle loss: When paired with proper protein intake and resistance exercise, intermittent fasting may assist sustain muscle mass. Fasting, in fact, may stimulate the creation of growth hormone, which aids in muscle maintenance and development.

4. Fasting Is Harmful to Women: While fasting may be appropriate for many women, individual requirements and circumstances must be considered. Some women may need to change their fasting schedules, particularly if they are pregnant, nursing, or have a medical condition.

5. Fasting Causes Nutrient Deficiencies: When performed with attention to balanced meals and nutrient-dense foods throughout eating windows, intermittent fasting is unlikely to create nutritional deficits. Indeed, it may aid in nutritional use and digestion.

6. Fasting Causes Overeating During Mealtimes: Fasting does not usually result in overeating if people practice mindful eating throughout their meal periods. It may even promote healthier eating habits and portion management.

7. To Fast, You Must Skip Breakfast: Intermittent fasting is adaptable, and you may set a fasting plan that works for you. Some people miss breakfast (as in the 16/8 approach), while others skip supper or select various fasting times.

8. Fasting Is Only for Losing Weight: While intermittent fasting may be an effective technique for weight reduction, its advantages extend beyond that. Fasting may benefit metabolic health, insulin sensitivity, inflammation reduction, and lifespan.

9. Fasting is appropriate for everyone: Intermittent fasting may not be appropriate for everyone, particularly those with severe medical issues, eating disorders, or who are on certain medicines.

10. Fasting Guarantees Quick Results: The effects of intermittent fasting differ from person to person. While some people may observe dramatic improvements, others will see slow development. The key to success is consistency and a comprehensive approach to health, which includes exercise and a well-balanced diet.

9 798868 019357